Paleo Diet
For Weight Loss
By M. Usman

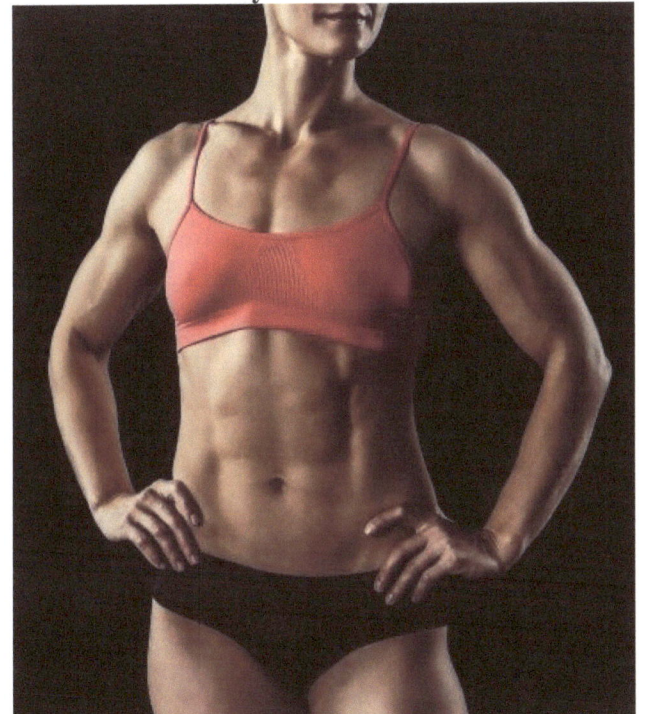

Health Learning Series

Mendon Cottage Books

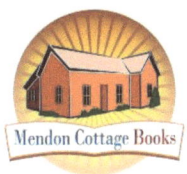

JD-Biz Publishing

Disclaimer

The information is this book is provided for informational purposes only. It is not intended to be used and medical advice or a substitute for proper medical treatment by a qualified health care provider. The information is believed to be accurate as presented based on research by the author.

The contents have not been evaluated by the U.S. Food and Drug Administration or any other Government or Health Organization and the contents in this book are not to be used to treat cure or prevent disease.

The author or publisher are not responsible for the use or safety of any diet, procedure or treatment mentioned in this book. The author or publisher is not responsible for errors or omissions that may exist.

Warning

The Book is for informational purposes only and before taking on any diet, treatment or medical procedure it is recommended to consult with your primary care provider.

Our books are available at

1. Amazon.com

2. Barnes and Noble

3. Itunes

4. Kobo

5. Smashwords

6. Google Play Books

Table of Contents

Paleo Diet – An Introduction

What is Paleo Diet?

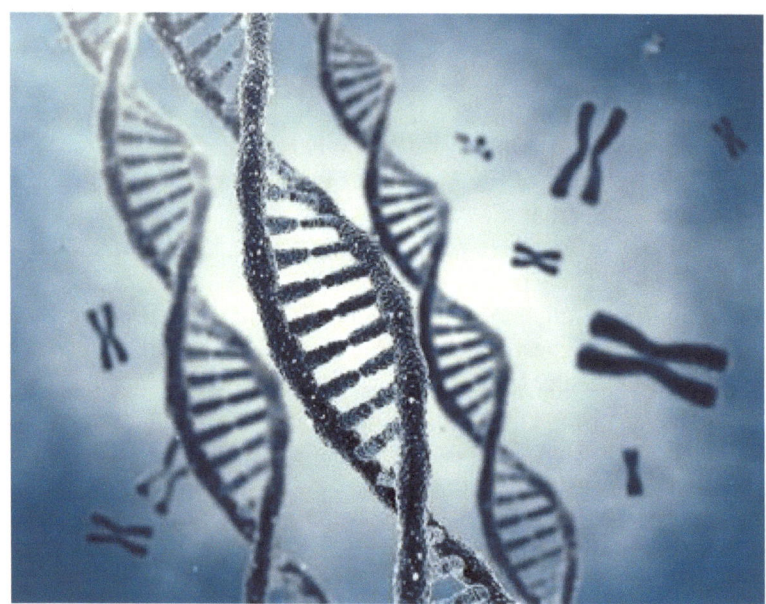

Basically, Paleo diet is a fancy word for caveman diet; it's what our ancestors used to consume tens of thousands of years ago when hunting was the only way to acquire food. The fundamental concepts behind the Paleo diet boil down to the genetic level. Simply put, our DNA has not significantly changed over the past 40 thousand years, and therefore, our bodies have not yet fully reformed to the contemporary, highly processed and artificial food items that are available in abundance nowadays. Thus the Paleo style of eating is the most biologically appropriate diet for us.

What can I eat?

Paleo diet includes anything that can be hunted or gathered. Clearly, hunting is not an option to acquire food nowadays but you can still obtain it from a supermarket, if of course the food was readily available during the Paleolithic period. Paleo diet includes and is not limited to meat, fish, vegetables, eggs, shellfish, tree nuts, roots, fruits, coconut palm sugar and raw honey.

Dairy, potatoes, processed oils, grains, legumes and sugars are to be avoided, along with salt and any drinks except water, coconut water and green tea. The diet of course eliminates any processed and readymade foods available today and is gluten free, largely due to the exclusion of grains.

What good will Paleo do for me?

As the Paleo diet is based entirely on whole foods, fresh fruits and vegetables and has lower amounts of sugar, sodium and manufactured foods than the average human diet; the human body can reap several benefits from it. By eliminating processed foods, which are often loaded with fats, as well as many other foods, people are likely to ingest fewer calories and therefore lose unwanted body weight.

Will Paleo Diet have any negative impact on my health?

As with any restrictive diet that eliminates complete food groups, there is always a risk of nutrient deficits. The Paleo diet excludes dairy products, which makes us vulnerable to calcium and vitamin D deficiencies, and grains, which may result in B vitamins and fiber deficiencies. These nutrients are imperative in the body for bone strength and a healthy digestive tract.

Do you have any evidence for your claims?

Of course I do. I am telling you now that the Paleo diet DOES work; but then again I know you wouldn't want to take my word for it because of the hugely commercialized and magnified diet plans all claiming to help you lose weight but not living up to their claim.

> I've been lucky. I haven't fallen into the "try every diet" trap. I've done a few, to be sure. Now I've found my diet home: the Paleo Diet. Since changing the diet and eating habits of my family to follow the wisdom and science behind the Paleo Diet, my husband, children and myself are leaner, not meaner, but certainly stronger and best of all, healthy and fit.

Jan A. Turning Leaf Touch

There is a building amount of evidence supporting a higher protein diet for weight loss and reduced risk of lifestyle disease. Similarly, there are also numerous studies that suggest that whole grains, legumes and low fat dairy have an effective place in a healthy diet, therefore, their addition in the current American Dietary Guidelines based on available research deemed to have sufficient strength to be considered reliable. Furthermore, research papers published by Dr. Loran Cordain claim that:

"A Paleolithic diet based on lean meat, fish, vegetables and fruit may be effective in the prevention and treatment of many common Western diseases that include and are in no way limited to cardiovascular diseases, insulin resistance, stroke and type 2 diabetes."

So, I challenge you to understand the Paleo diet and how it will help you lose weight if you do get on it and follow it.

Paleo Diet Weight Loss

Chapter # 1: Overview

Basically, your body is meant for storing extra calories instead of losing them. But what happens when if you consume more calories for a long period of time? The answer is very simple, you start gaining weight. When your diet is rich in calories i.e. rich in calories derived from simple carbs and saturated fats, your body's metabolic processes are overloaded and it's left with no other choice but to store extra calories in the form of fats. According to several researches if you consume more than 2500 calories each day, you eventually gain weight. So, Paleo diet being low in calories and using proteins and unsaturated fats (healthy fats) as the source of calories puts less strain on body's metabolic process. To put in simple words, Paleo diet helps lose weight both through burning extra fat and decreasing fat storage.

Chapter # 2: Under the Hood

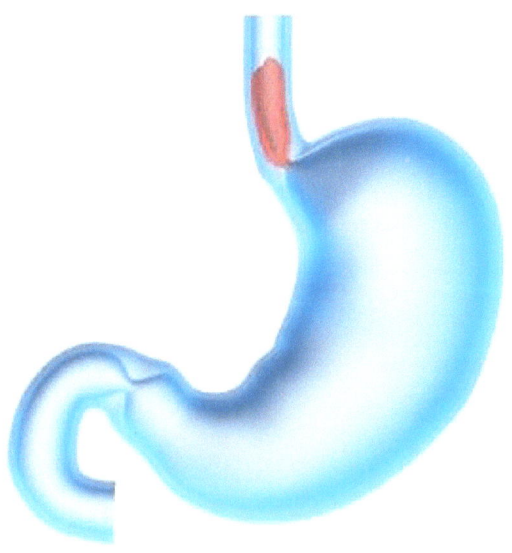

When you consume food that can be classified as Paleo Diet, two things are happening inside your body. First, the liver stores glucose by converting it into glycogen. Once you finish digesting all the carbs that you previously ate, the liver starts converting the stored glycogen back into glucose in the blood. Since the carbohydrate content of Paleo diet is very low, the glycogen stores run out very quickly. This is when your body is left with no other choice but to burn fats to produce energy. How does this happen? Your body breaks down fat cells and the liver manufactures ketones from these cells. The ketones now replace glucose as the fuel that burns in your cells. In nut shell, stored carbohydrates are replaced by stored fat as the main source of energy in your body.

To further get a hold of the concept as to how your body loses weight on the Paleo diet, you must consider the way the body uses sugar as fuel. To produce fuel from sugars, your body uses insulin. What part does insulin play in raising glucose levels? Insulin raises glucose and it does that by following basic ways:

- It generates new glucose by the breakdown of proteins
- It decreases the breakdown of glucose itself.

And when the glucose levels rise it diverts it to the fat storage pathway. It also keeps the body from burning stored fat. You must be getting the idea by now; it is the insulin that is the real culprit behind all this and as Paleo diet is low on carbohydrates insulin doesn't even get a chance to accumulate fat!

Chapter # 3: Paleo Diet, What and What not

You shouldn't be surprised to find a lack of packaged foods on the Paleo Diet menu. There were no grocery stores in the Stone Age, and if you're one of the 31 percent of Americans who eats more packaged foods than fresh foods in your daily diet, then maybe that's the only reason you're gaining weight and this habit of yours needs adjustment

Foods that are part of the Paleo Diet include the following:

- Lean red meats, game meats and organ meats
- Pork

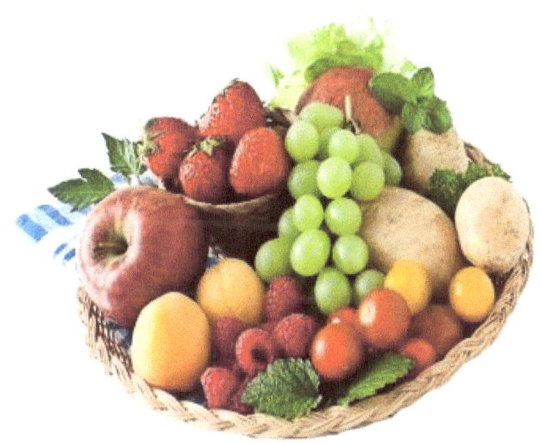

- Poultry
- Fish and shellfish

- Eggs
- Leafy and cruciferous vegetables
- Root vegetables
- Mushrooms
- Fruits
- Nuts

And in small amounts dried fruits, honey, coconut oil, olive oil, avocado oil and animal fats.

What's not allowed when following the diet?

- Grains (cereals such as barley, corn, oats, rice, rye and wheat)
- Beans or legumes
- Dairy products
- Salt
- Refined sugar
- Refined fats
- Canned or processed meats, as well as fatty meats
- Bacon
- Soda and fruit juices

Chapter # 4 : Is that it ?

Paleo diet is not just about eating the right type of food. Paleo Diet literally means "Caveman Diet". 10,000 years ago humans had to hunt in order to acquire food and hunting required a great deal of physical effort. These people didn't go to gyms but still had bodies like professional wrestlers. Of course, this type of approach can't be taken in today's world; but you can still make little changes in your life to get the most of Paleo diet. You can walk a couple of blocks instead of taking a taxi, run a mile or two during the weekends or if you have time and the resources, join a gym. You will get all the rewards of a normal person following Paleo Diet; you'll just get there faster. This is what Paleo Diet is truly about.

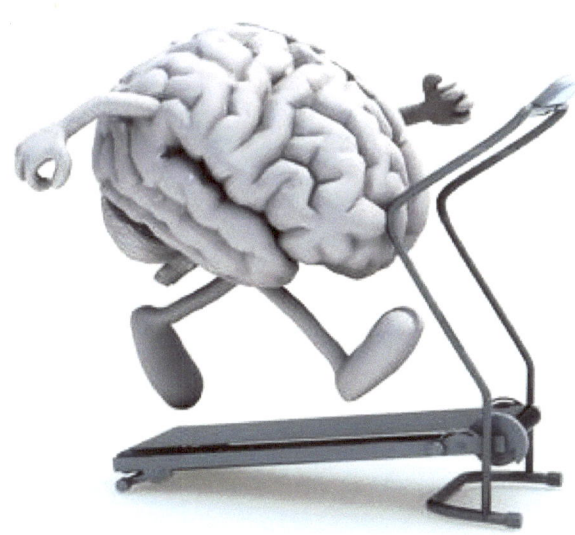

Paleo Diet vs. Other Diets

Chapter # 5: The world of diets

There are dozens of diet plans being advertised and even more are making their way into the scene. Many of these diets are purely a way to rip people off of their money and leave them tangled in a strange dietary jargon. But some diets, like the Paleo Diet have also established themselves successfully in the market, and are followed by millions of people worldwide. I have carefully prepared a list of diets that have gained popularity due to their effectiveness and in subsequent chapters I will be comparing each of them with the *Paleo Diet*.

1. Weight Watchers Diet:
2. Biggest Loser Diet:
3. Jenny Craig Diet:
4. Raw Food Diet:

I know they all have strange names but don't worry as I will be explaining each and every one of them.

Chapter # 6: Weight Watchers Diet

Followers of this particular diet can eat anything they want, the only limit being the quantity of the food they can eat. The amount that you can eat is controlled by a special "PointPlus" program that assigns every food a certain number of points based on the amount of carbohydrates, fat, fiber, calories and proteins in it. The points are also given on the basis of how hard the body has to work to burn a particular food. According to the program, foods that keep you from eating the longest are better than those that are just empty calories. Thus, a 200-calorie fruit smoothie will be a wiser choice than a 200-calorie iced coffee. To put in simple words, processed foods have a higher point value compared to whole foods as they contain a higher amount of carbohydrates, fats and comparatively low amount of proteins. A detailed list of point values of over 40,000 foods can be found on the Weight Watchers website (www.weightwatchers.com).

Before you go any further, I must tell you that apart from the cost of food, this diet is not free; you will need constant guidance about the diet plans and recipes and for this you would need to attend either weekly in-person meetings or register on their website. You can register, and use their services free of cost for a 3 month trial period.

How is it different from Pale Diet?

- The core principal behind the Paleo Diet is restrictions on specific food types whereas, the Weight Watchers Diet has no restriction on any specific food type but instead have to limit the size of their meals. This means Weight Watchers Diet gives its followers a larger variety to choose their food from.

- Followers of Paleo Diet have had great success in closing the doors to several life threatening diseases. There are numerous scientific evidences that support these claims. Unfortunately, this is not the case with Weight Watchers Diet. No doubt people have succeeded in clamping down cardiovascular diseases but there is no solid evidence to support these claims.

- There is a fair chance of you getting hungry if you don't choose the right meals. You can eat everything as long as it is confined to the Weight Watcher's *PointPlus* program. You would need to carry a *PointPlus* table and tally your meal before you can eat it. This can be quite a problem for those of us with little time. Paleo Diet in comparison does not restrict you in any way. A lot of meals in the Paleo Diet actually help start up the weight losing process.

- Since Weight Watchers Diet allows you to eat any kind of food, even simple carbs and saturated fats; it gets hard to cut down fat. Paleo, on the other hand confines you to specific foods. Therefore, you can obtain a flatter tummy faster if you follow the Paleo Diet.

- Weight Watchers Diet isn't free. You have to pay a certain amount to get access to *PointPlus* table, recipes and plans. But with Paleo Diet you're the boss. You can create your own dishes and just by keeping in mind the carbohydrate content of a food can take full control of your diet.

Chapter # 7: Biggest Loser Diet

This diet plan is a hybrid of low calorie food and physical activity; you'll have to do both or you'll go nowhere with it. This diet goes for six weeks in which you are bound to eat more "healthy foods" and do regular exercise. Nothing is off limits but the quantity is somewhat restricted, much like Weight Watchers diet. Each day, followers are required to eat four servings of vegetables and fruits, two of whole grains, three of protein. For extras, the Biggest Loser diet allows a maximum of 200 Calorie sugary desserts.

In order to follow the diet program, you will have to buy a "Biggest Loser" book. There are short and comprehensive books as well as bulky 30-Days one's too. You can choose the book of your liking. These books contain past success stories, tips for developing your menu and special food pyramids; All set to help you to sweat out some calories.

A lot of research has shown that sticking to this plan will certainly lead to weight loss and there's no rocket science behind how it works. It's simple; the Biggest Loser Diet places restrictions on what you eat and combines this with some pretty hectic exercise routines. Isn't that how Paleo Diet worked? Almost. Paleo Diet and Biggest Loser Diet are alike in a lot of ways but they are not the same.

How is it different from the Paleo Diet?

- Unlike the Paleo Diet, exercise is a big part of the Biggest Loser Diet. There are some pretty grueling routines that you must follow in order to make progress. If you don't follow these routines you won't make any progress. This is not the case with the Paleo Diet; exercise, is certainly a part of Paleo Diet too, but you would still lose weight even if you don't do it. Exercise helps you get there faster with Paleo Diet.

- There is no room for extras in the Paleo Diet. You are not allowed any "extras" when it comes to Paleo Diet and you must keep away from carbs for the plan to work.
- As physical activity is a huge part of the Biggest Loser Diet, its followers can beat more cardiovascular bad boys than those who follow the Paleo Diet.
- The cost of following this diet is certainly less than the Weight Watchers Diet but it's a tad more than the Paleo Diet too. You will have to invest in a gym in order to follow this diet.

Chapter # 8: Jenny Craig Diet

This specific diet plan is a multi-dimensional one; you'll have a personalized meal and exercise plan, plus a weekly counseling session with a Jenny Craig Diet consultant. Home cooked and restaurant meals will be largely off limits, prepackaged food will be delivered to you right at your doorstep. The diet will range from 1200 to 2000 calories per day. Your current weight, motivational and fitness level will be put under consideration when your specific diet and physical plan is being designed.

During the weekly counseling sessions you'll learn the amount of food you can eat, what a balanced meal is after you have graduated from this program, you can apply this knowledge. The initial registration fee at the time of writing of this book was 400 US dollars and a week's worth will cost you a 100.

According to a research, published in the health magazine, *Obesity* in 2007; it was found that those who stuck to the plan for a year lost 12 percent of their initial body weight, whereas those who gave up after the first month of the program lost just 1 percent. So it is quite evident that the Jenny Craig Diet works only on a long term basis so you'll have to stick to it to get the results.

How is it different from the Paleo Diet?

- Paleo Diet lets you be your own cook. This is not the case with the Jenny Craig Diet; Home-cooked meals are largely off-limits and you'll have to buy prepackaged meals from the Jenny Craig Company. The meals will be delivered right to your doorstep but if you are one of those who live a fast paced life you'll find yourself spending a lot of money on stocking these foods.

- Let's face it; the Jenny Craig Diet is a budget buster. Apart from the sharp registration fee you'll have to pay a steep price every time you order something. This is clearly not the case with the Paleo Diet.

- You'll have to attend weekly counseling sessions until you graduate as a "Jenny Craig expert". It's only after that you can prepare your own meals. Paleo Diet restricts you to specific food groups. You can cook any meal just by staying within those guidelines.

- Followers of Jenny Craig diet have had some cardiovascular benefits. There is still a lack of evidence to support these claims.

- Jenny Craig is effective in reducing your body weight but at a steep cost. The key to its success is the prepackaged food and psychological support, provided by the training counselors. Even though Paleo Diet plans don't have any guidance counselors, the success stories for those of you looking for a cost-effective solution to losing weight, the Jenny Craig diet is definitely not it.

Chapter # 9: Raw Food Diet

As simple as it sounds, this diet involves its followers to eat mostly fresh and uncooked food items throughout the day, every day until they have lost their desired weight. This diet does not include any physical activity but it's also doesn't forbid it. Exercise will help you shave extra pounds faster. The diet includes fresh fruits and vegetables, raw milk and its products, raw meat and every other food that isn't cooked above 115 degrees Fahrenheit. Advocates of this diet say that cooking eradicates most of the vitamins in food therefore, raw food is healthier and nourishing then cooked ones.

It is very likely that you will lose weight, provided you strictly follow the rules. Research suggests that those who follow the Raw Food diet tend to consume fewer calories and therefore weigh less than those who don't. In a study conducted and published by the Archives of Internal Medicine in 2005, "researchers compared 18 people on a strict raw food diet with 18 on a typical American diet. After 4 years, body mass index and mid-section fat were lower among those in the raw food group than those in the other group."

It is still unclear as to whether raw food diet has a positive cardiovascular effect. If followers of this diet heavily eat fruits and veggies they have a better chance to keep their cholesterol under control. There is also health risks linked to this diet; Undercooked meat, fish or eggs can lead to food poisoning. Furthermore, this diet is also inappropriate for infants and children due to its extreme restrictive nature.

How is it different from the Paleo Diet?

- Raw food diet plan restricts food types much in the same was as Paleo diet. But Paleo Diet doesn't advise you to eat uncooked food as does the Raw Food Diet plan. The Raw Food Diet claim that most of the nutrients are eliminated during cooking has no scientific evidence to support it. Actually, there are scientific proofs against this claim therefore; Paleo Diet is a much better option than Raw Food Diet.

- Weight loss is nearly guaranteed but at a cost: Eating raw food can lead to many unwanted diseases and germs taking refuge in your stomach. You won't be taking that big of a risk when following the Paleo Diet.

- Paleo Diet helps in controlling Type 2 Diabetes. There is still no good evidence that following the Raw Food Diet will bring your diabetes under control.

- It may cost a little more than Paleo Diet as this diet would require you to purchase some high end equipment such as blenders ranging from 300 to 500 US dollars. You may also require dehydrators that cost about 150 US dollars. Things don't get this complicated when following the Paleo Diet.

Chapter # 10: Diet Comparison Chart

	Simple Carbs	Sat Fat	Food Res	Cost Eff.*	Health Benefits	Lots of Homework	Extreme Exercise
Paleo	No	Yes	Yes	Yes	Yes	No	No
W.W.	Yes	Yes	No	No	Some	Yes	No
B.L.	Yes	Yes	Some	Some	Yes	Yes	Yes
J.C.	No	Yes	Yes	No	Yes	Yes	Yes
Raw	Some	Yes	Yes	No	Some	Yes	No

*Cost effectiveness excluding prices of food

Paleo Diet Menus

Unlike other diets that are making their way into the market, it is not a difficult task to make Paleo Diet a part of your life style. I will show you how painlessly you can switch to Paleo Diet without even noticing it.

Chapter # 11: Breakfast

- Easy Paleo Breakfast Ideas

  Here are some Paleo Breakfast Ideas for those of you in a hurry.

  1. Bacon, eggs, avocado, mushrooms & tomato.
  2. An omelet with your choice of meat, vegetables and of course – egg yolks as well as whites.
  3. Make a frittata with the veggies and meat of your choice.
  4. There's nothing like steak and eggs for breakfast!
  5. For a nutritionally dense Paleo Breakfast, chop up some chicken liver and scramble with eggs, onions and capsicum.
  6. Scrambled eggs mixed with diced bacon and avocado.
  7. Soft boiled eggs and wilted spinach.
  8. Make a soup with bone broth.
  9. Sweet potato, sardines and a poached egg.
  10. Try substitution bacon for skirt steak and serve with pumpkin.

No Time at all?

When you need a good, quick Paleo Breakfast and have no or little time to prepare a brunch, here are some ideas:

1. Paleo Breakfast Casserole – Put ingredients of your choice in a slow cooker and wake up to an instant hot breakfast.
2. Egg muffins – cook these up with your favorite veggies and meat in a big batch – and help yourself from the fridge all week.

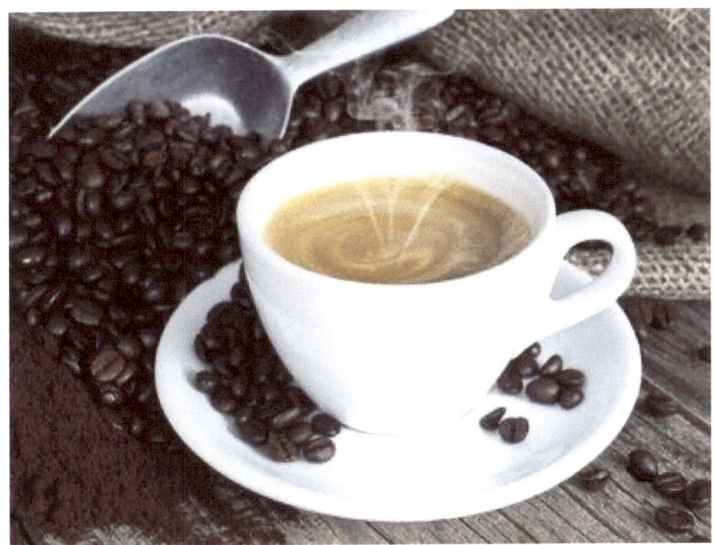

3. Make up a batch of salmon and zucchini croquettes to dig into all week.
4. Black Coffee.
5. Got a couple of minutes? Scramble an egg in a mug in the microwave.

Grab & Go

With no time to eat at home, here are some Paleo Breakfast ideas you can have while travelling:

---

1. Take a can of tuna/ mackerel/ kippers/ sardines and some pre-cut raw veggies.
2. Make a Paleo trail mix with your favorite nuts and dried fruit.
3. There's nothing wrong with beef jerky for breakfast!
4. Hard boiled eggs travel well and can be prepared in advance.
5. Coconut yoghurt.
6. Take a halved avocado and a spoon.

Cereal Substitutes

If you're missing your old crunchy breakfasts, there's a Paleo Diet grain-free equivalent for almost everything.

1. Make a Paleo cereal with nuts, berries and seeds in a bowls of almond milk.
2. Or try a Paleo cereal using dried fruit, seeds and nuts. Serve it with coconut milk and a pinch of cinnamon.
3. Paleo granola can be made up from your choice of nuts and served with coconut milk.
4. Make up banana bread with almond meal.

Something Fancy

If you have the time, there are some great ideas that are perfect for a special occasion. I very rarely use nuts and flours, but they are great for exceptional events.

1. Paleo pancakes with almond meal will take a tad more of your time, but in the end they're worth it.
2. Sweet potato pancakes.
3. Waffles can be made with coconut flour or almond meal and served with a berry sauce.

4. Raspberry Crepes made with coconut flour or almond meal served with fresh raspberries and whipped coconut cream – and a pinch of cinnamon.

5. A Paleo platter with a range of fruits, cold meats, pickles, olives, sundried tomatoes and blanched veggies.

6. Make bacon baskets using a cake case as a mould and bake eggs in them.

7. Stuff capsicum with salmon, mushroom and tomato and top with pine nuts.

8. Sliced onion wrapped with smoked salmon on a bed of lettuce.

9. Your favorite seafood & veggies.

10. Serve scrambled eggs in an orange half.

No Eggs!

For those of you who don't have a thing for eggs. Here are some egg free Paleo Breakfast Ideas:

1. Kippers and dried figs.

2. Pan fried zucchini served with guacamole.

3. Stuffed portabella mushrooms.

4. Sautee minced beef, greens, onions and carrots.

5. Sausages with sauerkraut & stir fried veggies.

6. Trout with mushrooms and tomato.

7. Fry kidneys and serve with broccoli.

Paleo Vegetarian Options

If you're a vegan, don't worry we have a menu for you too:

1. Poached eggs and sweet potato (or even yam) hash browns.

2. Sauté some greens, squeeze on some lemon and add an egg.

3. Fry eggs in a capsicum (bell pepper) ring or onion ring.

4. Steamed broccoli with sweet potatoes.

5. Mash up a hardboiled egg with avocados.

Fruit Friendly?

It is a good practice to minimize fruit intake, when on a Paleo Diet, due to its high sugar content. Still, if you want some fruit, you got it:

1. A nice simple fruit salad – served with whipped coconut cream.

2. Even easier – a piece of fruit and a few berries.

3. Make a warm fruit custard with eggs & coconut milk on the stove. Add some nutmeg, cinnamon, berries a banana and nuts for your pleasure.

4. Chop up a kiwi fruit in coconut cream.

Drinkable Breakfasts

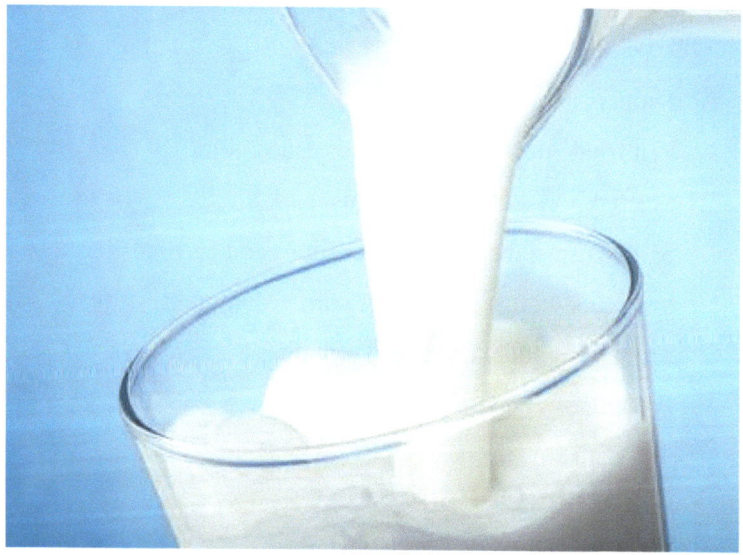

There are some good drinkable options too. Just be sure to add in some coconut oil and enjoy your breakfast drink!

1. Green smoothies; try adding in Kale and spinach for a vitamin boast.
2. Make an anti-oxidant berry smoothie with coconut milk.
3. A veggie juice with carrots, coconut milk, celery and broccoli.
4. A banana smoothie made with frozen bananas, coconut milk and almond butter.

Chapter #12 : Lunch

- Leftovers?

  If you've got access to a fridge and microwave, look no further as your options are countless; you can make stews, soups, Paleo chili and casseroles, freeze them and simply heat them at lunch times.

- Brown-Bag Lunches?

  For many of us, kitchen facilities aren't available and eating out isn't an option at lunchtime. So what can you put in a Paleo Packed Lunch? These are some suggestions from which you can pick the food of your choice:

  1. Make kebabs with your choice of meat and vegetables on sticks.
  2. Take in cold meat and veggies and pour over a hot bone broth from a thermos just before serving.
  3. A salad with meat, avocado, eggs, leaves, vegetables, nuts and seeds of your choice. Try lemon juice, extra virgin olive oil, and balsamic vinegar or crushed avocado for the dressing.
  4. Olives.
  5. Lettuce wraps, instead of bread. Use the lettuce instead of bread loaves.
  6. Invest in good thermos and bring in a hot ready to eat soup or stew straight to your work.
  7. Bag up last night's leftovers.
  8. Make up a crust less quiche or fritella.
  9. Blanch some veggies.
  10. Raw veggies with almond butter or guacamole dip.

---

11. Breadless sandwiches using cold meat or flat capsicum instead of bread.

12. Hard boiled eggs.

Chapter # 13: Dinner

Chicken Paleo Dinner

There are numerous options with chicken. Some of them are listed below.

1. Thai green curry.
2. Chicken Fajitas.
3. Chicken casserole.
4. Chicken Kebabs.
5. Bacon wrapped chicken breasts.
6. Roast chicken.
7. Chicken salad with mango.
8. Lemon chicken in the slow cooker.
9. Jerk chicken.
10. Quick & easy chicken curry.

Fish Paleo Dinner

Fish is enriched with a goodness of Omega 3 so there's no reason to avoid it.

1. Salmon burgers.
2. Paleo Sushi using nori wraps and cauliflower rice.
3. Pan seared tuna with lime and steamed veggies.
4. Smoked haddock omelette.
5. Chilli crab.
6. Salt & pepper squid.
7. Shrimp salad.
8. Chowder.
9. Baked trout & roasted vegetables.

10. Seared scallops.

Lamb Paleo Dinner

Lamb sounds delicious doesn't it?

1. Shepherd's pie topped with sweet potato mash.

2. Lamb shanks with cauliflower rice.

3. Lamb skewers.

4. Slow roasted leg of lamb.

5. Lamb tagine.

6. Lamb chops and mint sauce.

7. Lamb burgers served with a Greek salad.

Winter Paleo Diet Dinners

Something comforting for cold winter nights!

1. Bone broth.

2. Mushroom soup.

Conclusion

If there's one sentence that can conclude this book, it's that Losing weight and starting a better life is not an impossible thing; all you need is determination and someone to point you in the right direction. We have provided you with the latter; all you have to do is to have faith in yourself. Following the guidelines provided in this book, you can start a better life, a healthier life, and one where you're not at the risk of a heart attack or a stroke, one where you can live life to the fullest

Photo References

All images licensed by fotolia.com

Obst undGemüse

© PhotoSG - Fotolia.com

Kaffee

© jogyx - Fotolia.com

milk pouring into glass

© Nitr - Fotolia.com

Dna double helix molecules and chromosomes

© nobeastsofierce - Fotolia.com

Cooked Beef Roast

© portokalis - Fotolia.com

human brain on a running machine

© fabioberti.it - Fotolia.com

Heart attack of a businessman

© Nolight - Fotolia.com

Finger grabbing buffalo chicken wing

© Cappi Thompson - Fotolia.com

Cooked Beef Roast

© portokalis - Fotolia.com

References

1. Walter Voegtlin: The Stone age diet based on in-depth study of Human ecology and diet of man (1975) – CHAPTER 15: A 20th Century Stone age diet (http://www.mitodascalorias.com/wp-content/uploads/2013/06/Voegtlin_1975_The_Stone_Age_Diet.pdf)

2. Wikipedia's definition of Paleolithic diet (http://en.wikipedia.org/wiki/Paleolithic_diet)

3. Walter Voegtlin: The Stone age diet based on in-depth study of Human ecology and diet of man (1975) (http://www.mitodascalorias.com/wp-content/uploads/2013/06/Voegtlin_1975_The_Stone_Age_Diet.pdf)

4. Boyd Eaton, Loren Cordain, Staffan Lindeberg: Evolutionary Health Promotions: A consideration of common counterarguments. December, 2001. (http://thepaleodiet.com/wp-content/uploads/2012/04/Counter-Arguments_Paper.pdf)

5. Boyd Eaton: Paleolithic nutrition – A consideration of its nature and current implications 1985 (http://www.ncbi.nlm.nih.gov/pubmed/2981409?dopt=Abstract)

6. Gary Foster et al. A randomized trial of a Low Carbohydrate diet for Obesity.
   (http://inspire.stat.ucla.edu/unit_15/NEJM2082.pdf)

7. Staffan Lindeberg et al. Apparent absence of stroke and ischaemic heart disease in a traditional Melanesian island: a clinical study in Kitava.
   (http://onlinelibrary.wiley.com/doi/10.1111/j.1365-2796.1993.tb00986.x/abstract;jsessionid=7F1EEC9B23FCAD9333A2D12078313A4C.d02t01)

8. Loren Cordain and John Friel: The Paleo diet for athletes.
   (http://www.trainingbible.com/pdf/Paleo_for_Athletes_Cliff_Notes.pdf)

9. Dr. John McDougall: The Starch Solution
   (http://www.drmcdougall.com/store_starch_solution.html)

10. Dr. Denis Murphy: People, plants and genes – The Story of Crops and Humanity.
    (http://www.oxfordscholarship.com/view/10.1093/acprof:oso/9780199207145.001.0001/acprof-9780199207145)

11. Katherine Milton: Hunter-gatherer diets – a different perspective
    (http://ajcn.nutrition.org/content/71/3/665.long)

12. Alexander Strohle et al.: Carbohydrates and the diet-atherosclerosis connection--more between earth and heaven. Comment on the article "The atherogenic potential of dietary carbohydrate". (http://scholar.qsensei.com/content/1321gb http://www.ncbi.nlm.nih.gov/pubmed/16997359)

13. US. News and World Reports 2012 – Best overall diets (http://health.usnews.com/best-diet/best-overall-diets)

Author Bio

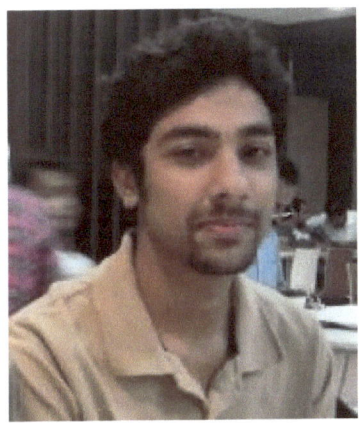

Muhammad Usman is a distinguished medical graduate of Allama iqbal medical college (AIMC). He is a professional writer who has been in the field for more than 4 years. During this time he has produced 10,000+ articles, blogs and eBooks on various niches related to diseases, health, fitness, nutrition and well being. He is a regular contributor to several journals related to medicine and surgery. He is the editor of several journals and newspapers.

Check out some of the other JD-Biz Publishing books

Gardening Series on Amazon

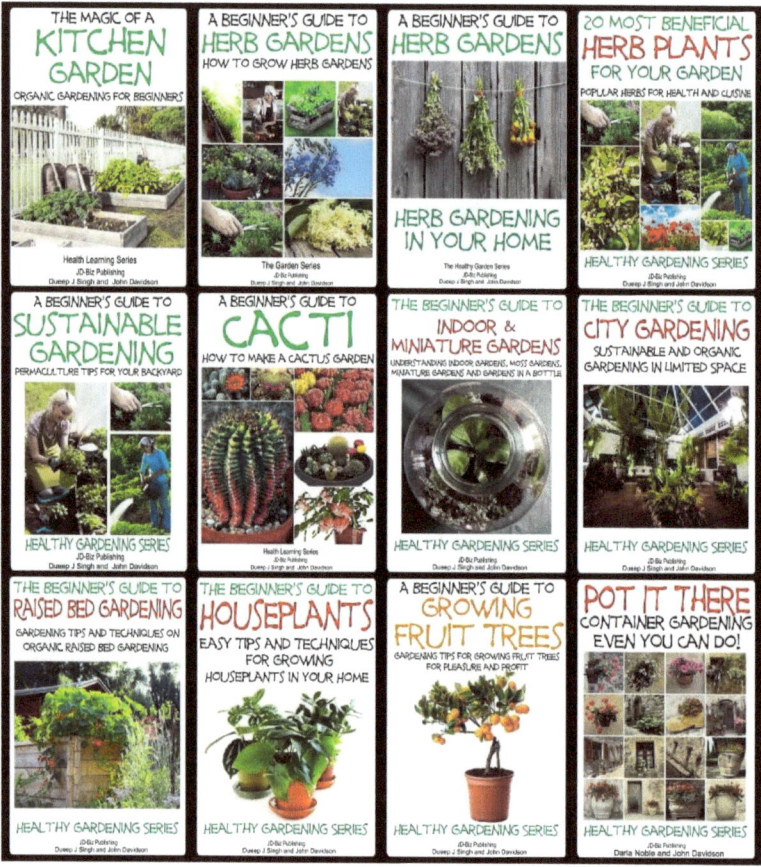

Health Learning Series

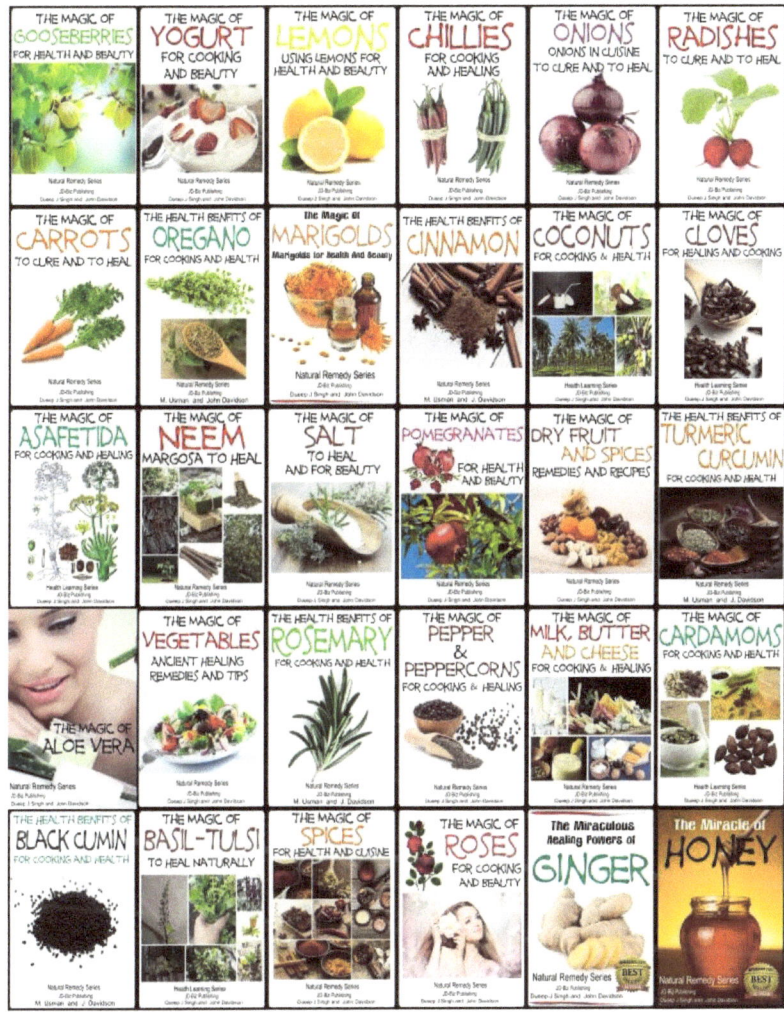

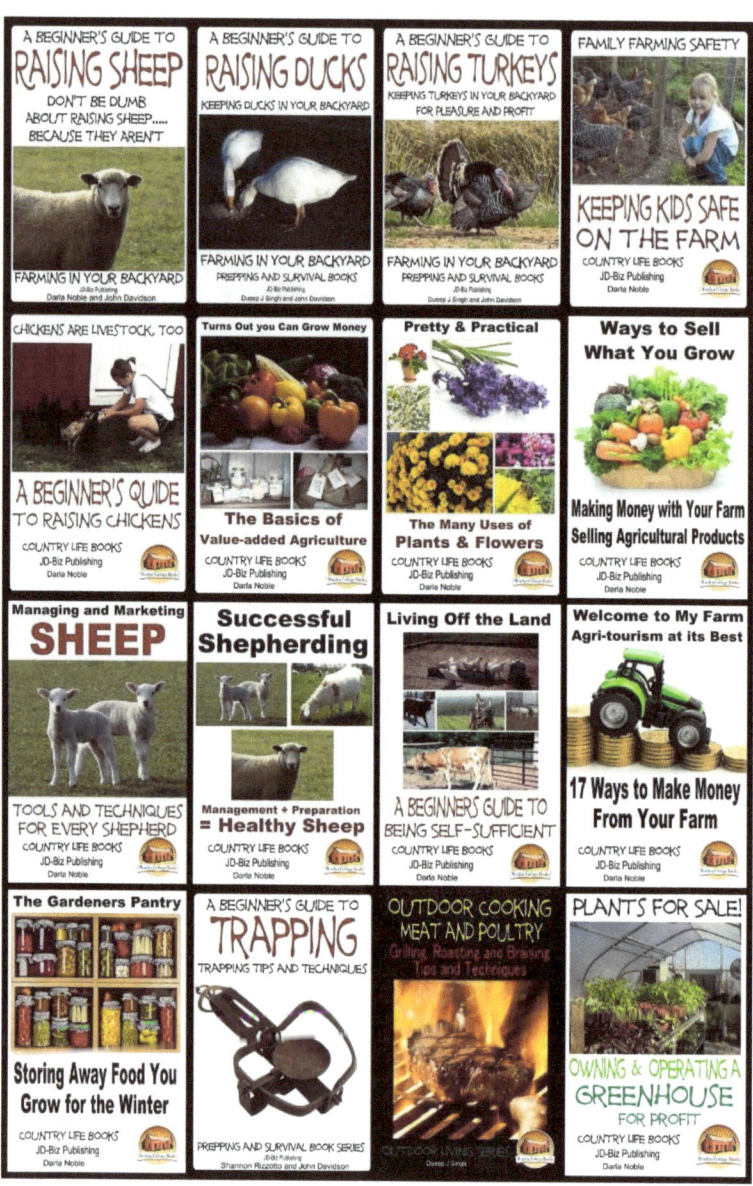

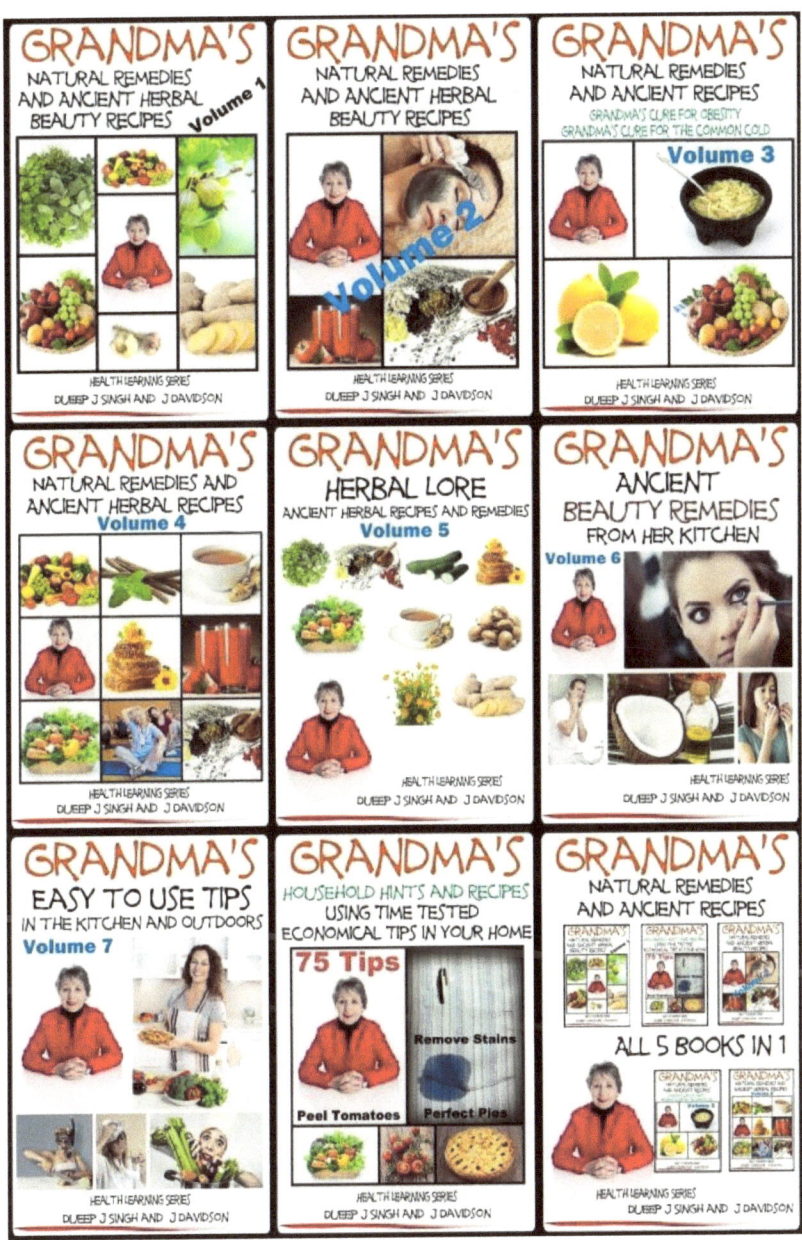

Health Learning Series

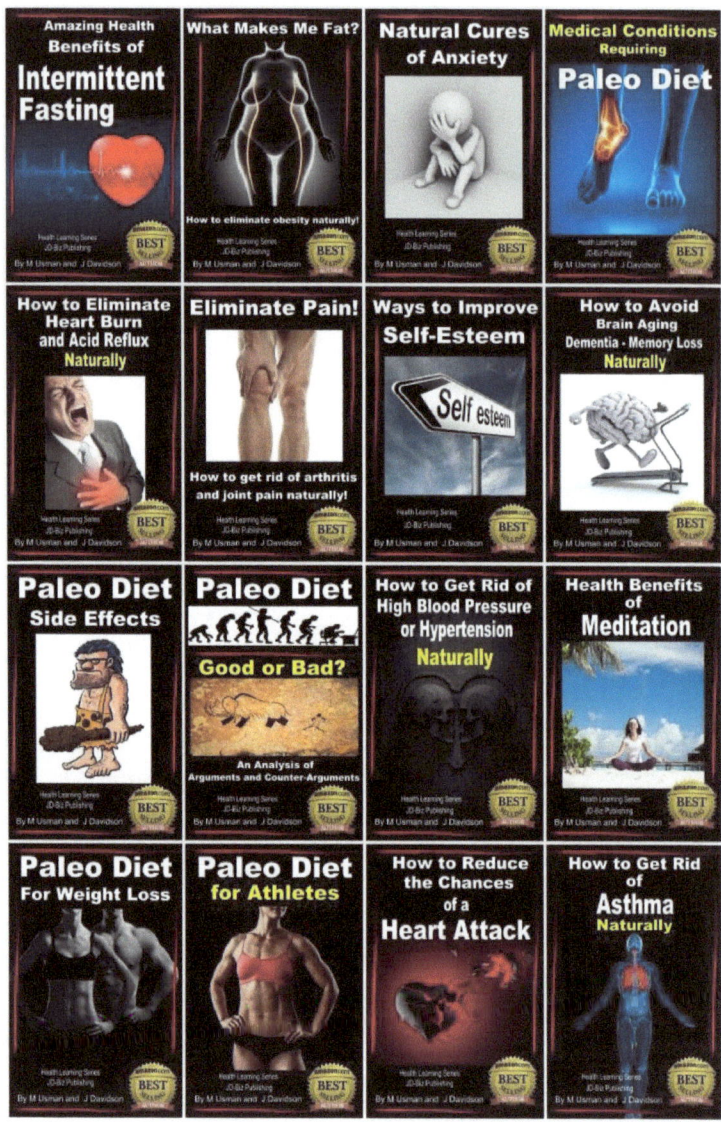

Amazing Animal Book Series

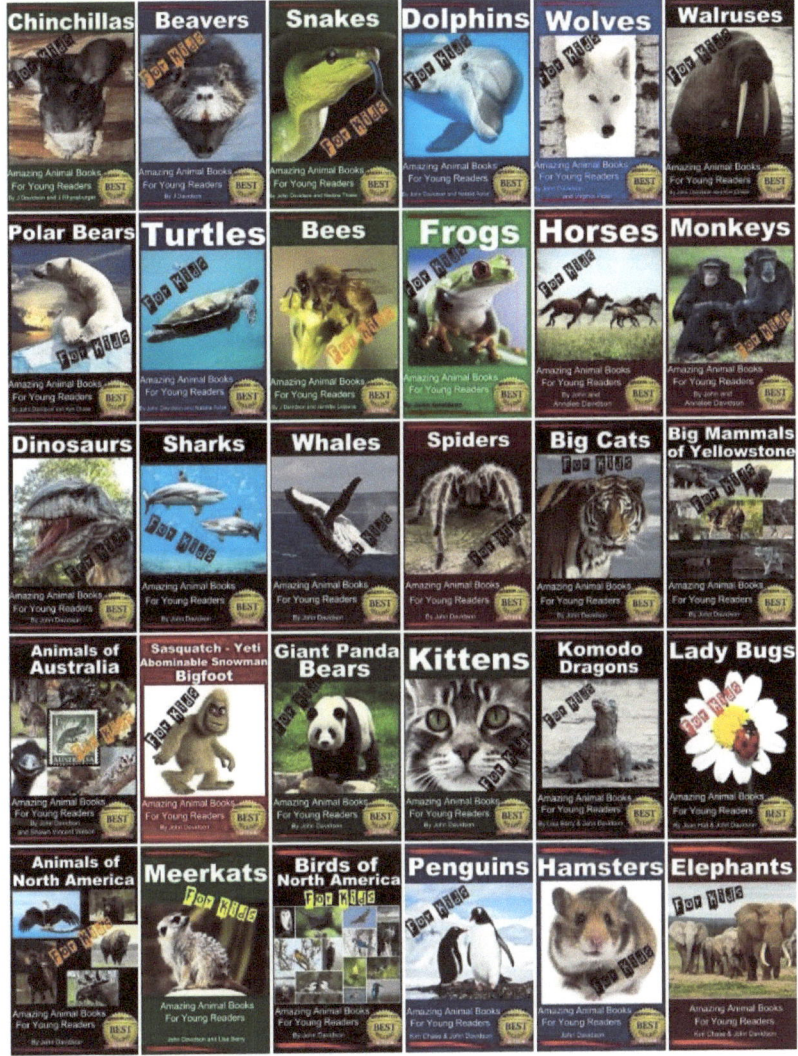

Learn To Draw Series

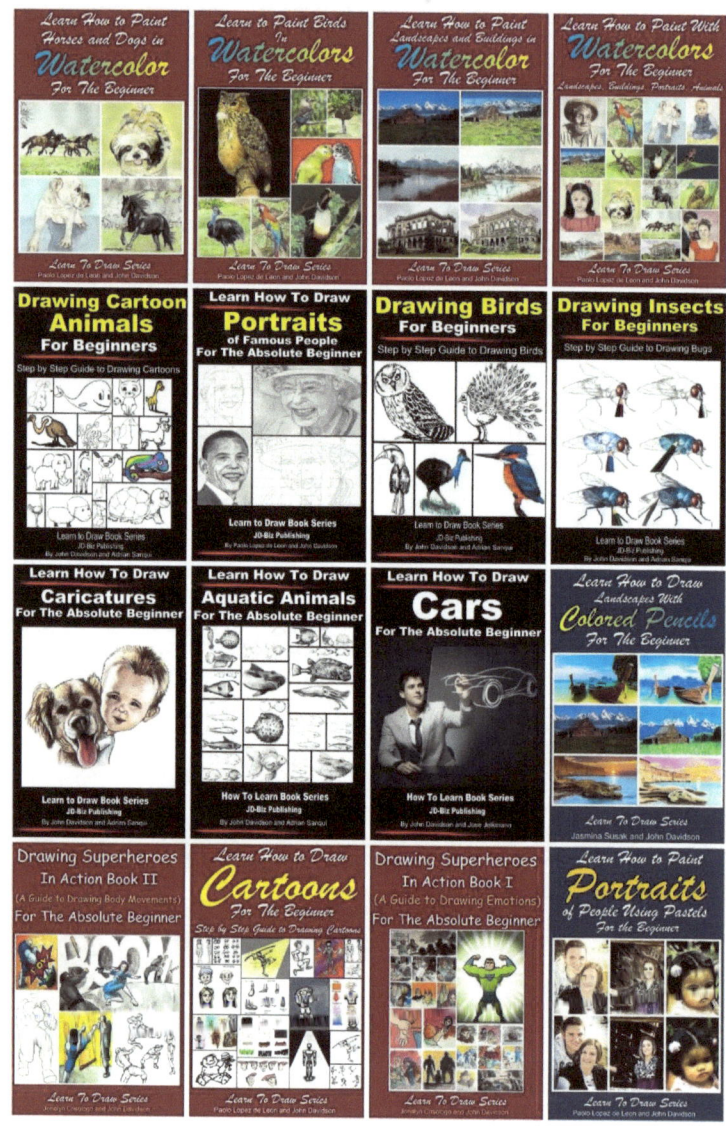

How to Build and Plan Books

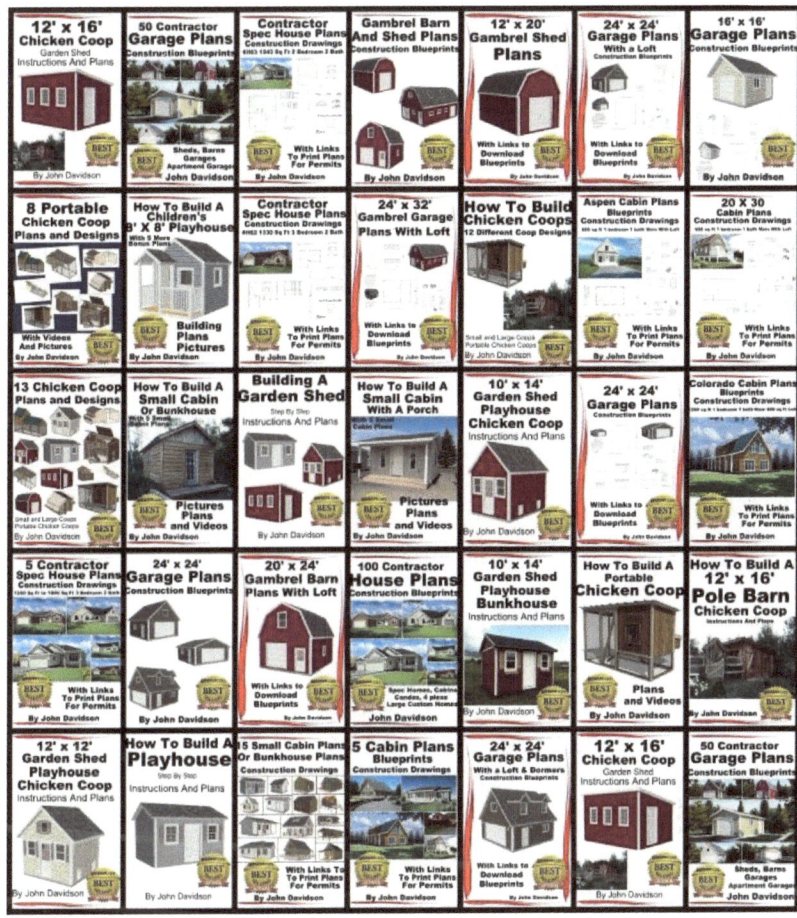

Entrepreneur Book Series

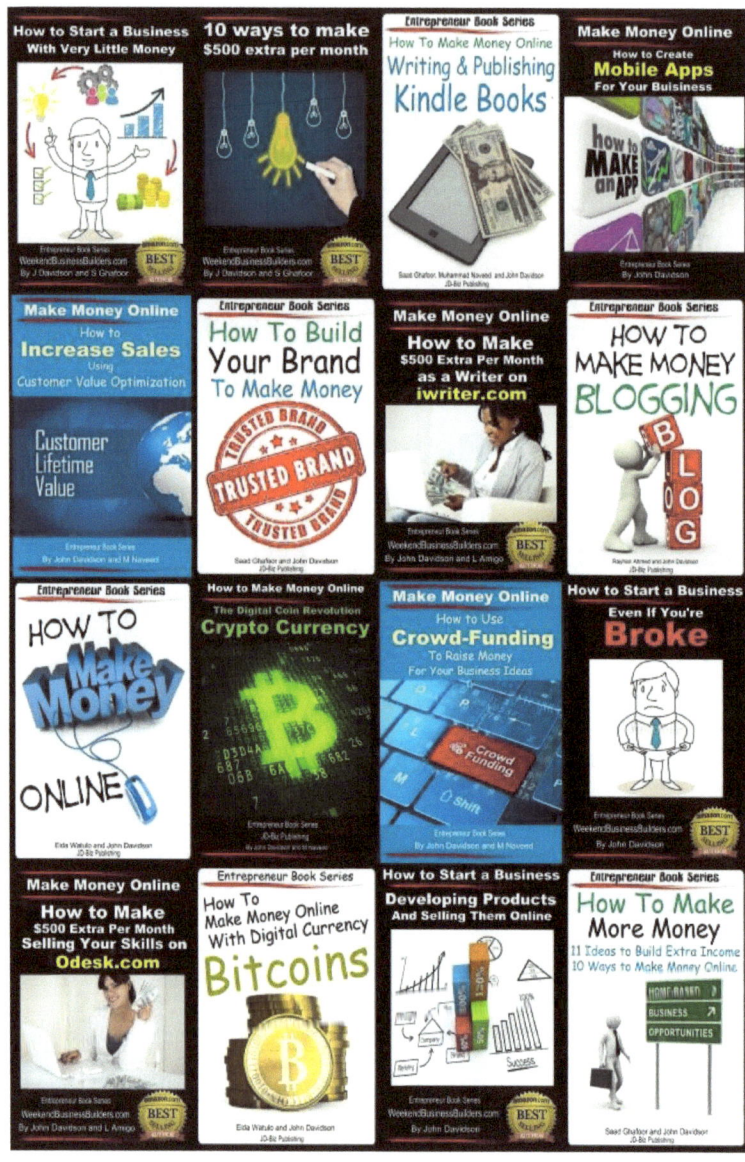

Our books are available at

1. Amazon.com
2. Barnes and Noble
3. Itunes
4. Kobo
5. Smashwords
6. Google Play Books

Download Free Books!
http://MendonCottageBooks.com

Publisher

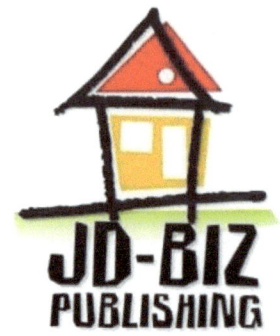

JD-Biz Corp

P O Box 374

Mendon, Utah 84325

http://www.jd-biz.com/

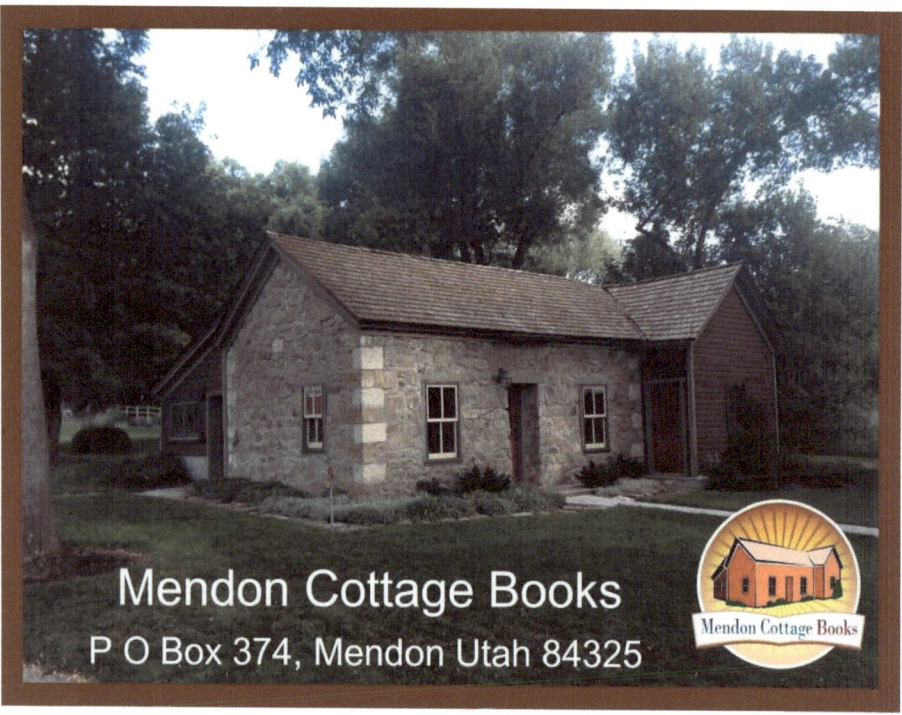

www.ingramcontent.com/pod-product-compliance
Lightning Source LLC
Chambersburg PA
CBHW050833290526
45792CB00001B/376